C0001787774

# The Ultimate Smoothie Collection for Beginners

*Boost your Metabolism and your Health with these Quick, Easy and Delicious Smoothies*

**Elisa Brooks**

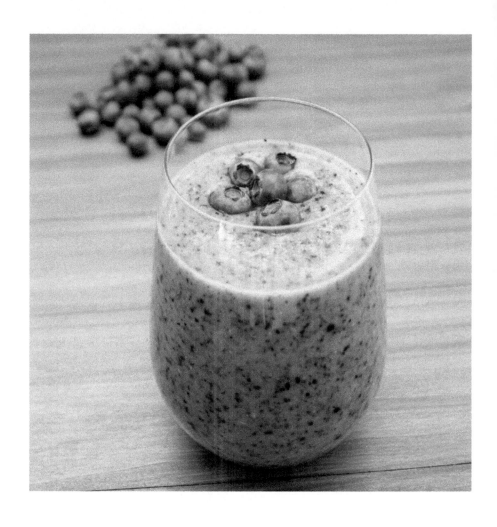

# Table of Contents

# Minty Green Smoothie

## Ingredients

➤ ½ of avocado; peeled, pitted, and chopped

➤ 1 cup fresh kale leaves

➤ ½ of small cucumber, peeled and chopped

➤ ¼ cup fresh mint leaves

➤ 1 tablespoon almond butter

➤ 1 tablespoon fresh lemon juice

➤ 1¼ cups unsweetened almond milk

➤ ½ cup ice cubes

## How to Prepare

1.    Add all the ingredients in a high-power blender and pulse until creamy.

2.    Pour the smoothie into two glasses and serve immediately.

Preparation time: 10 minutes Total time: 10 minutes Servings: 2

## Nutritional Values

➤ Calories 195

➤ Total Fat 15.2 g

➤ Saturated Fat 2.4 g

➤ Cholesterol 0 mg

➤ Sodium 137 mg

➤ Total Carbs 13.8 g

➤ Fiber 6 g

➤ Sugar 2 g

➤ Protein 5.1 g

# Spiced Smoothie

## Ingredients

➤ 2 tablespoons chia seeds

➤ 1 tablespoon ground turmeric

➤ 1 teaspoon ground cinnamon

➤ 1 teaspoon ground ginger

➤ ¼ teaspoon ground cardamom

➤ Pinch of ground black pepper

➤ 2 tablespoons MCT oil

➤ 2 teaspoons stevia powder

➤ 1¾ cups unsweetened almond milk

➤ ¼ cup ice cubes

## How to Prepare

1.   Add all the ingredients in a high-power blender and pulse until creamy.

2.   Pour the smoothie into two glasses and serve immediately.

Preparation time: 10 minutes Total time: 10 minutes
Servings: 2

## Nutritional Values

➢ Calories 183

➢ Total Fat 20 g

➢ Saturated Fat 14.6 g

➢ Cholesterol 0 mg

➢ Sodium 159 mg

➢ Total Carbs 8.7 g

➢ Fiber 4.9 g

➢ Sugar 0.2 g

➢ Protein 2.8 g

# Pineapple & Turmeric Smoothie

## Ingredients

➤ 1½ cups pineapple, chopped

➤ 1 (1-inch) piece fresh ginger, peeled and chopped

➤ 1 teaspoon ground turmeric

➤ 1 teaspoon natural immune support

➤ 1 teaspoon chia seeds

➤ 1 cup cold green tea

➤ ½ cup ice, crushed

## How to Prepare

1.    Add all the ingredients in a high-power blender and pulse until creamy.

2.    Pour the smoothie into two glasses and serve immediately.

Preparation time: 10 minutes Total time: 10 minutes Servings: 2

## Nutritional Values

➢ Calories 104

➢ Total Fat 1.1 g

➢ Saturated Fat 0.1 g

➢ Cholesterol 0 mg

➢ Sodium 12 mg

➢ Total Carbs 24.9 g

➢ Fiber 2.9 g

➢ Sugar 18.8 g

➢ Protein 1.3 g

# Watermelon & Strawberry Smoothie

## Ingredients

➤ 1½ cups fresh watermelon, seeded and cubed

➤ 1 cup frozen strawberries

➤ ½ of frozen banana, peeled and sliced

➤ 1 tablespoon hemp seeds

➤ 2 tablespoons fresh lime juice

➤ 1 cup unsweetened almond milk

## How to Prepare

1. Add all the ingredients in a high-power blender and pulse until creamy.

2. Pour the smoothie into two glasses and serve immediately.

Preparation time: 10 minutes Total time: 10 minutes Servings: 2

## Nutritional Values

➤ Calories 126

- ➤ Total Fat 3.9 g

- ➤ Saturated Fat 0.4 g

- ➤ Cholesterol 0 mg

- ➤ Sodium 93 mg

- ➤ Total Carbs 22.2 g

- ➤ Fiber 3 g

- ➤ Sugar 14.1 g

- ➤ Protein 3.2 g

# Grapefruit & Pineapple Smoothie

## Ingredients

➢ 3 grapefruit; peeled, seeded, and chopped

➢ ½ cup frozen pineapple chunks

➢ 1½ cups unsweetened almond milk

➢ ¼ cup ice cubes

## How to Prepare

1. Add all the ingredients in a high-power blender and pulse until creamy.

2. Pour the smoothie into two glasses and serve immediately.

Preparation time: 10 minutes Total time: 10 minutes Servings: 2

## Nutritional Values

➢ Calories 112

➢ Total Fat 2.9 g

➢ Saturated Fat 0.3 g

➤ Cholesterol 0 mg

➤ Sodium 136 mg

➤ Total Carbs 22.4 g

➤ Fiber 3.4 g

➤ Sugar 17.5 g

➤ Protein 2.2 g

# Berries Yogurt Smoothie

## Ingredients

➤ 1½ cups frozen mixed berries

➤ ½ teaspoon vanilla extract

➤ 1 cup plain yogurt

➤ 1 cup fresh orange juice

➤ ¼ cup ice cubes

## How to Prepare

1. Add all the ingredients in a high-power blender and pulse until creamy.

2. Pour the smoothie into two glasses and serve immediately.

Preparation time: 10 minutes Total time: 10 minutes Servings: 2

## Nutritional Values

➤ Calories 206

➤ Total Fat 2.1 g

- ➤ Saturated Fat 1.3 g

- ➤ Cholesterol 7 mg

- ➤ Sodium 87 mg

- ➤ Total Carbs 34.4 g

- ➤ Fiber 4 g

- ➤ Sugar 26.7 g

- ➤ Protein 8.6 g

# Cherry & Blueberry Smoothie

## Ingredients

➤ 1¼ cups frozen blueberries

➤ 1 cup frozen unsweetened cherries

➤ 1 small banana, peeled and slice

➤ 6 ounces fat-free plain yogurt

➤ 1 cup unsweetened almond milk

## How to Prepare

1. Add all the ingredients in a high-power blender and pulse until creamy.

2. Pour the smoothie into two glasses and serve immediately.

Preparation time: 10 minutes Total time: 10 minutes Servings: 2

## Nutritional Values

➤ Calories 203

➤ Total Fat 2.3 g

➤ Saturated Fat 0.2 g

➤ Cholesterol 2 mg

➤ Sodium 156 mg

➤ Total Carbs 43 g

➤ Fiber 5.5 g

➤ Sugar 24.7 g

➤ Protein 6.5 g

# Pineapple & Cucumber Smoothie

## Ingredients

➢   1 cup pineapple, chopped

➢   1 cucumber, peeled and chopped

➢   4 Medjool dates, pitted

➢   2 tablespoons fresh lemon juice

➢   1½ cups filtered water

## How to Prepare

1.   Add all the ingredients in a high-power blender and pulse until creamy.

2.   Pour the smoothie into two glasses and serve immediately.

Preparation time: 10 minutes Total time: 10 minutes Servings: 2

## Nutritional Values

➢   Calories 193

➢   Total Fat 0.4 g

- ➤ Saturated Fat 0.2 g

- ➤ Cholesterol 0 mg

- ➤ Sodium 7 mg

- ➤ Total Carbs 49.6 g

- ➤ Fiber 5.1 g

- ➤ Sugar 39.2 g

- ➤ Protein 3.1 g

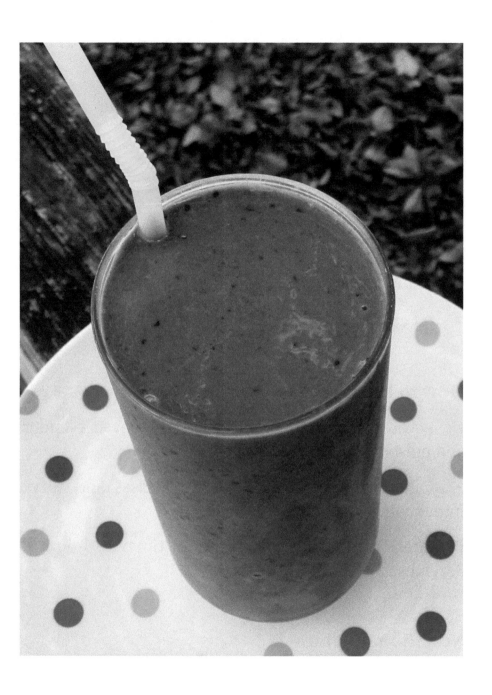

# Carrot & Pineapple Smoothie

## Ingredients

➤ 2 cups carrot, peeled and chopped

➤ 2 cups pineapple chunks

➤ 1 tablespoon fresh ginger, grated

➤ 1½ tablespoons fresh lemon juice

➤ 1 cup ice cubes

## How to Prepare

1. Add all the ingredients in a high-power blender and pulse until creamy.

2. Pour the smoothie into two glasses and serve immediately.

Preparation time: 10 minutes Total time: 10 minutes Servings: 2

## Nutritional Values

➤ Calories 139

➤ Total Fat 0.5 g

- ➤ Saturated Fat 0.2 g

- ➤ Cholesterol 0 mg

- ➤ Sodium 81 mg

- ➤ Total Carbs 34.6 g

- ➤ Fiber 5.4 g

- ➤ Sugar 22 g

- ➤ Protein 2.1 g

# Cranberry & Grapefruit Smoothie

## Ingredients

➢ ½ cup fresh cranberries

➢ 2 grapefruit; peeled, seeded, and sectioned

➢ 1 frozen banana, peeled and sliced

➢ 1 tablespoon agave nectar

➢ ¾ cup fresh orange juice

➢ ½ cup unsweetened almond milk

➢ ¼ cup ice cubes

## How to Prepare

1. Add all the ingredients in a high-power blender and pulse until creamy.

2. Pour the smoothie into two glasses and serve immediately.

Preparation time: 10 minutes Total time: 10 minutes Servings: 2

## Nutritional Values

- Calories 190

- Total Fat 1.4 g

- Saturated Fat 0.2 g

- Cholesterol 0 mg

- Sodium 46 mg

- Total Carbs 44.5 g

- Fiber 4.9 g

- Sugar 32.5 g

- Protein 2.3 g

# Date & Almond Smoothie

## Ingredients

➤ 1 cup Medjool dates, pitted and chopped

➤ ½ cup almonds, chopped

➤ 1½ cups unsweetened almond milk

➤ ¼ cup ice cubes

## How to Prepare

1. Add all the ingredients in a high-power blender and pulse until creamy.

2. Pour the smoothie into two glasses and serve immediately.

Preparation time: 10 minutes Total time: 10 minutes Servings: 2

## Nutritional Values

➤ Calories 418

➤ Total Fat 14.9 g

➤ Saturated Fat 1.2 g

- Cholesterol 0 mg

- Sodium 137 mg

- Total Carbs 73.4 g

- Fiber 10.8 g

- Sugar 57.4 g

- Protein 8 g

# Chocolaty Peanut Butter Smoothie

## Ingredients

➤ ¼ cup creamy peanut butter

➤ 2 tablespoons cacao powder

➤ 8–10 drops liquid stevia

➤ 1 cup heavy cream

➤ 1 cup unsweetened almond milk

➤ ¼ cup ice cubes

## How to Prepare

1. Add all the ingredients in a high-power blender and pulse until creamy.

2. Pour the smoothie into two glasses and serve immediately.

Preparation time: 10 minutes Total time: 10 minutes Servings: 2

## Nutritional Values

➤ Calories 429

- ➢ Total Fat 41.2 g

- ➢ Saturated Fat 18 g

- ➢ Cholesterol 82 mg

- ➢ Sodium 261 mg

- ➢ Total Carbs 11.5 g

- ➢ Fiber 3.9 g

- ➢ Sugar 3.1 g

- ➢ Protein 10.8 g

# Banana Peanut Butter Smoothie

## Ingredients

➤ 2 cups frozen bananas, peeled and sliced

➤ 2 tablespoons all-natural peanut butter

➤ ½ tablespoon ground flax seeds

➤ 1 teaspoon vanilla extract

➤ ½ cup plain Greek yogurt

➤ 1 cup unsweetened almond milk

## How to Prepare

1. Add all the ingredients in a high-power blender and pulse until creamy.

2. Pour the smoothie into two glasses and serve immediately.

Preparation time: 10 minutes Total time: 10 minutes Servings: 2

## Nutritional Values

➤ Calories 312

- ➢ Total Fat 11.6 g

- ➢ Saturated Fat 2.5 g

- ➢ Cholesterol 4 mg

- ➢ Sodium 138 mg

- ➢ Total Carbs 43.3 g

- ➢ Fiber 5.9 g

- ➢ Sugar 24 g

- ➢ Protein 11 g

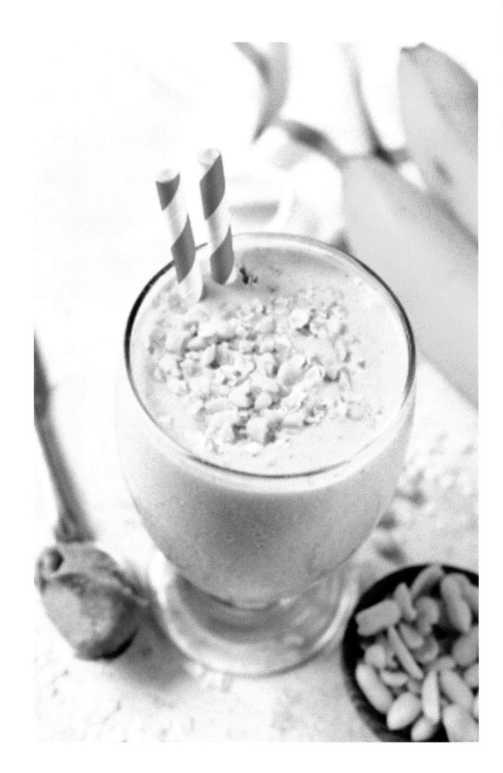

# Raspberry Peanut Butter Smoothie

## Ingredients

➤ 1 banana, peeled and sliced

➤ 2 cups fresh raspberries

➤ 2 tablespoons peanut butter

➤ 1 tablespoon honey

➤ 1½ cups unsweetened almond milk

➤ ¼ cup ice cubes

## How to Prepare

1. Add all the ingredients in a high-power blender and pulse until creamy.

2. Pour the smoothie into two glasses and serve immediately.

Preparation time: 10 minutes Total time: 10 minutes Servings: 2

## Nutritional Values

➤ Calories 278

➤ Total Fat 11.6 g

➤ Saturated Fat 1.8 g

➤ Cholesterol 0 mg

➤ Sodium 140 mg

➤ Total Carbs 41.3 g

➤ Fiber 11.3 g

➤ Sugar 22.3 g

➤ Protein 7.9 g

# Creamy Blackberry Smoothie

## Ingredients

➤ 1 cup fresh blackberries

➤ ½ cup heavy whipping cream

➤ ½ cup cream cheese, softened

➤ ½ tablespoon coconut oil

➤ 3–5 drops liquid stevia

➤ 1 cup chilled water

## How to Prepare

1. Add all the ingredients in a high-power blender and pulse until creamy.

2. Pour the smoothie into two glasses and serve immediately.

Preparation time: 10 minutes Total time: 10 minutes Servings: 2

## Nutritional Values

➤ Calories 366

- ➤ Total Fat 35.1 g

- ➤ Saturated Fat 22.6 g

- ➤ Cholesterol 105 mg

- ➤ Sodium 184 mg

- ➤ Total Carbs 9.3 g

- ➤ Fiber 3.8 g

- ➤ Sugar 3.7g

- ➤ Protein 6 g

# Berries Cream Smoothie

## Ingredients

➤ 1 cup mixed fresh berries

➤ 1 tablespoon MCT oil

➤ ½ teaspoon vanilla extract

➤ 3–5 drops liquid stevia

➤ ¾ cup heavy whipping cream

➤ 1 cup unsweetened almond milk

➤ ¼ cup ice cubes

## How to Prepare

1.    Add all the ingredients in a high-power blender and pulse until creamy.

2.    Pour the smoothie into two glasses and serve immediately.

Preparation time: 10 minutes Total time: 10 minutes Servings: 2

## Nutritional Values

➤ Calories 268

➤ Total Fat 25.7 g

➤ Saturated Fat 17.5 g

➤ Cholesterol 62 mg

➤ Sodium 108 mg

➤ Total Carbs 10.9 g

➤ Fiber 3 g

➤ Sugar 2.2 g

➤ Protein 1.9 g

# Kiwi & Melon Smoothie

## Ingredients

➤ 2 kiwi fruit, peeled and chopped

➤ 1 cup honeydew melon, peeled and chopped

➤ ½ teaspoon fresh ginger, chopped

➤ 1½ scoops unsweetened protein powder

➤ ½ tablespoon fresh lime juice

➤ 1¾ cups fresh grape juice

➤ ¼ cup ice cubes

## How to Prepare

1.  Add all the ingredients in a high-power blender and pulse until creamy.

2.  Pour the smoothie into two glasses and serve immediately.

Preparation time: 10 minutes Total time: 10 minutes Servings: 2

## Nutritional Values

➤ Calories 314

➤ Total Fat 1.8 g

➤ Saturated Fat 0.1 g

➤ Cholesterol 0 mg

➤ Sodium 217 mg

➤ Total Carbs 53.8 g

➤ Fiber 3.4 g

➤ Sugar 48.5 g

➤ Protein 22.7 g

# Sweet Potato Smoothie

## Ingredients

➤ 1 medium frozen banana, peeled and sliced

➤ 1 cup sweet potato puree

➤ 1 teaspoon fresh ginger, chopped

➤ ½ tablespoon flax seeds meal

➤ 1 tablespoon almond butter

➤ ¼ teaspoon ground turmeric

➤ ¼ teaspoon ground cinnamon

➤ 1 cup unsweetened almond milk

➤ ¼ cup fresh orange juice

➤ ¼ cup ice cubes

## How to Prepare

1.    Add all the ingredients in a high-power blender and pulse until creamy.

2.    Pour the smoothie into two glasses and serve immediately.

Preparation time: 10 minutes Total time: 10 minutes
Servings: 2

## Nutritional Values

➤ Calories 242

➤ Total Fat 7.5 g

➤ Saturated Fat 0.7 g

➤ Cholesterol 0 mg

➤ Sodium 128 mg

➤ Total Carbs 41.7 g

➤ Fiber 7.1 g

➤ Sugar 16.7 g

➤ Protein 5.7 g

# Pumpkin & Banana Smoothie

## Ingredients

➤   ¾ cup pumpkin puree

➤   2 medium frozen bananas, peeled and sliced

➤   ½ teaspoon pumpkin pie spice

➤   1 scoop unsweetened whey protein powder

➤   4–6 drops liquid stevia

➤   ½ cup plain Greek yogurt

➤   1 cup unsweetened almond milk

## How to Prepare

1.   Add all the ingredients in a high-power blender and pulse until creamy.

2.   Pour the smoothie into two glasses and serve immediately.

Preparation time: 10 minutes Total time: 10 minutes Servings: 2

## Nutritional Values

➤ Calories 259

➤ Total Fat 3.7 g

➤ Saturated Fat 1.1 g

➤ Cholesterol 4 mg

➤ Sodium 271 mg

➤ Total Carbs 40 g

➤ Fiber 6.3 g

➤ Sugar 21.8 g

➤ Protein 19 g

# Matcha Spinach & Pineapple Smoothie

## Ingredients

➤ ½ cup frozen pineapple

➤ 1 cup fresh baby spinach

➤ ½ of avocado; peeled, pitted, and chopped

➤ 2 tablespoons honey

➤ 1 tablespoon coconut oil

➤ 1 teaspoon matcha green tea powder

➤ ½ cup fresh orange juice

➤ 1 cup unsweetened almond milk

## How to Prepare

1. Add all the ingredients in a high-power blender and pulse until creamy.

2. Pour the smoothie into two glasses and serve immediately.

Preparation time: 10 minutes Total time: 10 minutes Servings: 2

## Nutritional Values

➢ Calories 297

➢ Total Fat 18.6 g

➢ Saturated Fat 8.1 g

➢ Cholesterol 0 mg

➢ Sodium 107 mg

➢ Total Carbs 35 g

➢ Fiber 5 g

➢ Sugar 26.8 g

➢ Protein 2.6 g

# Chocolate Smoothie

## Ingredients

➤ 2 cups fresh spinach

➤ ½ cup fresh blueberries

➤ 2 Medjool dates, pitted

➤ 1–2 tablespoons raw cacao nibs

➤ 1 tablespoon ground chia seeds

➤ 1 cup unsweetened cashew milk

➤ ¼ cup ice cubes

## How to Prepare

1.    Add all the ingredients in a high-power blender and pulse until creamy.

2.    Pour the smoothie into two glasses and serve immediately.

Preparation time: 10 minutes Total time: 10 minutes Servings: 2

## Nutritional Values

➤ Calories 148

➤ Total Fat 4.1 g

➤ Saturated Fat 1.1 g

➤ Cholesterol 0 mg

➤ Sodium 106 mg

➤ Total Carbs 27.4 g

➤ Fiber 6.8 g

➤ Sugar 17.9 g

➤ Protein 3.3 g

# Coffee Chia Smoothie

## Ingredients

➤   1 tablespoon chia seeds

➤   1 tablespoon MCT oil

➤   ½ teaspoon ground cinnamon

➤   ½ cup heavy whipping cream

➤   12 ounces cold brewed coffee

➤   ½ cup unsweetened almond milk

## How to Prepare

1.    Add all the ingredients in a high-power blender and pulse until creamy.

2.    Pour the smoothie into two glasses and serve immediately.

Preparation time: 10 minutes Total time: 10 minutes Servings: 2

## Nutritional Values

➤   Calories 181

- Total Fat 20.3 g

- Saturated Fat 14.1 g

- Cholesterol 41 mg

- Sodium 60 mg

- Total Carbs 3.3 g

- Fiber 1.8 g

- Sugar 0 g

- Protein 1.8 g

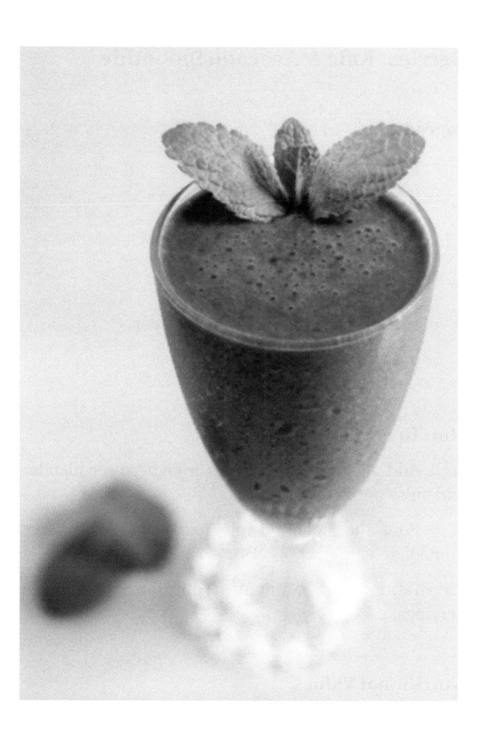

# Berries, Kale & Avocado Smoothie

## Ingredients

➢ 1 cup frozen blueberries

➢ 1 cup fresh kale leaves

➢ ½ of avocado

➢ 3 Medjool dates, pitted

➢ ½ teaspoon green spirulina powder

➢ 2 cups soy milk

## How to Prepare

1. Add all the ingredients in a high-power blender and pulse until creamy.

2. Pour the smoothie into two glasses and serve immediately.

Preparation time: 10 minutes Total time: 10 minutes Servings: 2

## Nutritional Values

➢ Calories 389

- ➤ Total Fat 14.3 g

- ➤ Saturated Fat 2.6 g

- ➤ Cholesterol 0 mg

- ➤ Sodium 149 mg

- ➤ Total Carbs 58.6 g

- ➤ Fiber 9.5 g

- ➤ Sugar 38.5 g

- ➤ Protein 12 g

# Berries & Pomegranate Smoothie

## Ingredients

➤ 2 cups mixed fresh berries

➤ 2 tablespoons chia seeds

➤ 1¼ cups fresh pomegranate juice

➤ ¾ cup filtered water

## How to Prepare

1.  Add all the **ingredients** in a high-power blender and pulse until creamy.

2.  Pour the smoothie into two glasses and serve immediately.

Preparation time: 10 minutes Total time: 10 minutes Servings: 2

## Nutritional Values

➤ Calories 209

➤ Total Fat 3 g

➤ Saturated Fat 0.2 g

- ➤ Cholesterol 0 mg

- ➤ Sodium 13 mg

- ➤ Total Carbs 45 g

- ➤ Fiber 7.5 g

- ➤ Sugar 31.3 g

- ➤ Protein 2.5 g

# Blueberry & Avocado Smoothie

## Ingredients

➤ 2 cups fresh blueberries

➤ 1 large banana, peeled and sliced

➤ 1 small avocado; peeled, pitted, and chopped

➤ 1 tablespoon chia seeds

➤ 1 cup fresh cranberry juice

➤ ¼ cup ice cubes

## How to Prepare

1. Add all the ingredients in a high-power blender and pulse until creamy.

2. Pour the smoothie into two glasses and serve immediately.

Preparation time: 10 minutes Total time: 10 minutes Servings: 2

## Nutritional Values

➤ Calories 304

- ➤ Total Fat 12 g

- ➤ Saturated Fat 2.5 g

- ➤ Cholesterol 0 mg

- ➤ Sodium 5 mg

- ➤ Total Carbs 47.9 g

- ➤ Fiber 12.3 g

- ➤ Sugar 25 g

- ➤ Protein 3.7 g

# Raspberry & Egg Smoothie

## Ingredients

➤ 1 frozen banana, peeled and sliced

➤ 1½ cups fresh raspberries

➤ 2 eggs

➤ 1 tablespoon honey

➤ ½ cup plain yogurt

➤ 1 cup unsweetened almond milk

## How to Prepare

1.   Add all the ingredients in a high-power blender and pulse until creamy.

2.   Pour the smoothie into two glasses and serve immediately.

Preparation time: 10 minutes Total time: 10 minutes Servings: 2

## Nutritional Values

➤ Calories 259

- Total Fat 7.7 g

- Saturated Fat 2.2 g

- Cholesterol 167 mg

- Sodium 196 mg

- Total Carbs 38.8 g

- Fiber 8.1 g

- Sugar 24.6 g

- Protein 11.3 g

# Green Pumpkin Seed Smoothie

## Ingredients

➤ 2 apples; peeled, cored, and chopped

➤ 1 cup frozen blueberries

➤ 2 cups fresh baby spinach

➤ ¼ cup pumpkin seeds

➤ 1½ tablespoons flax seeds

➤ 1 tablespoon raw wheat germ

➤ 4–6 drops liquid stevia

➤ 1½ cups fresh apple juice

## How to Prepare

1.   Add all the ingredients in a high-power blender and pulse until creamy.

2.   Pour the smoothie into two glasses and serve immediately.

Preparation time: 10 minutes Total time: 10 minutes Servings: 2

## Nutritional Values

➤ Calories 384

➤ Total Fat 10.9 g

➤ Saturated Fat 1.9 g

➤ Cholesterol 0 mg

➤ Sodium 38 mg

➤ Total Carbs 69.7 g

➤ Fiber 10.8 g

➤ Sugar 49.1 g

➤ Protein 8.4 g

# Lemony Blackberry Smoothie

## Ingredients

➤    2 cups frozen blackberries

➤    1 small banana, peeled and sliced

➤    2 tablespoons fresh lime juice

➤    1 tablespoon honey

➤    1 teaspoon lime zest, grated

➤    ½ cup plain yogurt

➤    1 cup light coconut milk

## How to Prepare

1.    Add all the ingredients in a high-power blender and pulse until creamy.

2.    Pour the smoothie into two glasses and serve immediately.

Preparation time: 10 minutes Total time: 10 minutes Servings: 2

## Nutritional Values

➤ Calories 259

➤ Total Fat 7.6 g

➤ Saturated Fat 5.2 g

➤ Cholesterol 4 mg

➤ Sodium 83 mg

➤ Total Carbs 44.6 g

➤ Fiber 9.1 g

➤ Sugar 29.2 g

➤ Protein 6.1 g

# Cherry Smoothie

## Ingredients

➤ 2 cup frozen cherries, pitted

➤ 1 medium frozen banana, peeled and sliced

➤ 1½ cups unsweetened almond milk

## How to Prepare

1. Add all the ingredients in a high-power blender and pulse until creamy.

2. Pour the smoothie into two glasses and serve immediately.

Preparation time: 10 minutes Total time: 10 minutes Servings: 2

## Nutritional Values

➤ Calories 154

➤ Total Fat 3.5 g

➤ Saturated Fat 0.5 g

➤ Cholesterol 0 mg

- ➤ Sodium 137 mg

- ➤ Total Carbs 32.1 g

- ➤ Fiber 4.8 g

- ➤ Sugar 21.2 g

- ➤ Protein 2.8 g

# Turmeric Fruity Smoothie

## Ingredients

➤ 2 medium frozen bananas, peeled and sliced

➤ 1 cup frozen mango cubes

➤ 1 teaspoon fresh turmeric, peeled and grated

➤ 1 teaspoon fresh ginger, peeled and grated

➤ 1 tablespoon hemp seeds

➤ ¼ teaspoon vanilla extract

➤ 2 cups soy milk

## How to Prepare

1.    Add all the ingredients in a high-power blender and pulse until creamy.

2.    Pour the smoothie into two glasses and serve immediately.

Preparation time: 10 minutes Total time: 10 minutes Servings: 2

## Nutritional Values

➤ Calories 316

➤ Total Fat 6.9 g

➤ Saturated Fat 0.9 g

➤ Cholesterol 0 mg

➤ Sodium 128 mg

➤ Total Carbs 58.4 g

➤ Fiber 6.3 g

➤ Sugar 35.6 g

➤ Protein 11.4 g

# Kiwi & Avocado Smoothie

## Ingredients

➤ 1 kiwi, peeled and chopped

➤ 1 small avocado; peeled, pitted, and chopped

➤ 1 cup cucumber, peeled and chopped

➤ 2 cups fresh baby kale

➤ ¼ cup fresh mint leaves

➤ 2 cups filtered water

➤ ¼ cup ice cubes

## How to Prepare

1.   Add all the ingredients in a high-power blender and pulse until creamy.

2.   Pour the smoothie into two glasses and serve immediately.

Preparation time: 10 minutes Total time: 10 minutes Servings: 2

## Nutritional Values

➤ Calories 185

➤ Total Fat 11.4 g

➤ Saturated Fat 2.4 g

➤ Cholesterol 0 mg

➤ Sodium 38 mg

➤ Total Carbs 20.3 g

➤ Fiber 7 g

➤ Sugar 4.6 g

➤ Protein 4.2 g

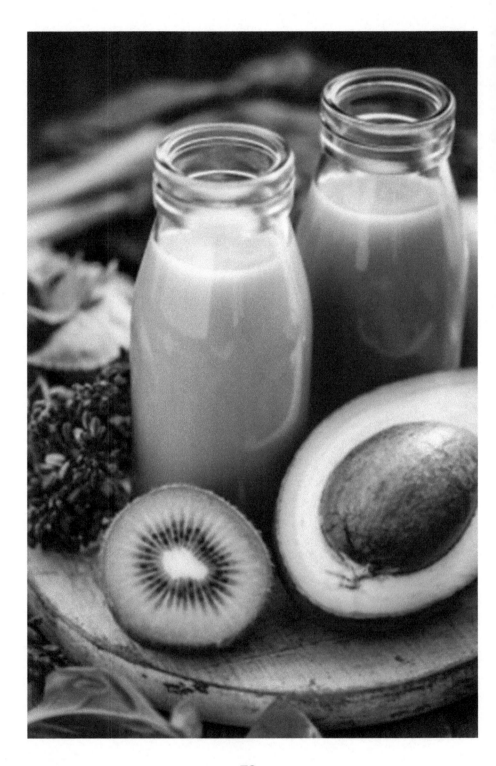

# Matcha Chia Seed Smoothie

## Ingredients

➤ 2 tablespoons chia seeds

➤ 2 teaspoons matcha green tea powder

➤ ½ teaspoon fresh lime juice

➤ 6–8 drops liquid stevia

➤ ¼ cup coconut yogurt

➤ 1¼ cups unsweetened coconut milk

➤ ¼ cup ice cubes

## How to Prepare

1. Add all the ingredients in a high-power blender and pulse until creamy.

2. Pour the smoothie into two glasses and serve immediately.

Preparation time: 10 minutes Total time: 10 minutes Servings: 2

## Nutritional Values

➤ Calories 276

➤ Total Fat 24.5 g

➤ Saturated Fat 20.2 g

➤ Cholesterol 1 mg

➤ Sodium 54 mg

➤ Total Carbs 8.2 g

➤ Fiber 2.5 g

➤ Sugar 4.8 g

➤ Protein 4.9 g

# Zucchini & Spinach Smoothie

## Ingredients

➢ 1 small zucchini, peeled and sliced

➢ ¾ cup fresh spinach, chopped

➢ 1 teaspoon ground cinnamon

➢ 4–6 drops liquid stevia

➢ 1½ cups unsweetened almond milk

➢ ½ cup ice cubes

## How to Prepare

1. Add all the ingredients in a high-power blender and pulse until creamy.

2. Pour the smoothie into two glasses and serve immediately.

Preparation time: 10 minutes Total time: 10 minutes Servings: 2

## Nutritional Values

➢ Calories 45

- ➢ Total Fat 2.8 g

- ➢ Saturated Fat 0.3 g

- ➢ Cholesterol 0 mg

- ➢ Sodium 150 mg

- ➢ Total Carbs 4.8 g

- ➢ Fiber 2.3 g

- ➢ Sugar 1.1 g

- ➢ Protein 1.8 g

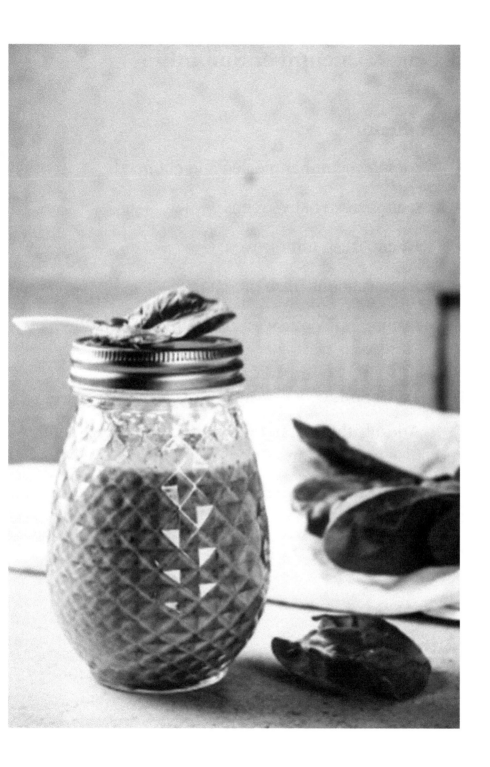

# Greens & Cucumber Smoothie

## Ingredients

➤ 1 large cucumber, peeled and chopped

➤ 2 cups fresh baby greens

➤ ¼ cup fresh mint leaves

➤ 2 tablespoons fresh lime juice

➤ 2 cups chilled unsweetened almond milk

## How to Prepare

1.  Add all the ingredients in a high-power blender and pulse until creamy.

2.  Pour the smoothie into two glasses and serve immediately.

Preparation time: 10 minutes Total time: 10 minutes Servings: 2

## Nutritional Values

➤ Calories 72

➤ Total Fat 3.8 g

- ➢ Saturated Fat 0.4 g

- ➢ Cholesterol 0 mg

- ➢ Sodium 190 mg

- ➢ Total Carbs 9.2 g

- ➢ Fiber 2.9 g

- ➢ Sugar 2.9 g

- ➢ Protein 2.7 g

# Avocado & Mint Smoothie

## Ingredients

➤ 1 avocado; peeled, pitted, and chopped

➤ 12–14 fresh large mint leaves

➤ 2 tablespoons fresh lime juice

➤ ½ teaspoon vanilla extract

➤ 1½ cups unsweetened almond milk

➤ ¼ cup ice, crushed

## How to Prepare

1. Add all the ingredients in a high-power blender and pulse until creamy.

2. Pour the smoothie into two glasses and serve immediately.

Preparation time: 10 minutes Total time: 10 minutes Servings: 2

## Nutritional Values

➤ Calories 214

- Total Fat 18.5 g

- Saturated Fat 2.6 g

- Cholesterol 0 mg

- Sodium 45 mg

- Total Carbs 11.7 g

- Fiber 8.9 g

- Sugar 0.4 g

- Protein 3.3 g

# Green Veggies Smoothie

## Ingredients

➤ 1 cup fresh spinach

➤ ¼ cup broccoli florets, chopped

➤ ¼ cup green cabbage, chopped

➤ ½ of small green bell pepper, seeded and chopped

➤ 8–10 drops liquid stevia

➤ 2 cups chilled water

## How to Prepare

1. Add all the ingredients in a high-power blender and pulse until creamy.

2. Pour the smoothie into two glasses and serve immediately.

Preparation time: 10 minutes Total time: 10 minutes Servings: 2

## Nutritional Values

➤ Calories 19

- Total Fat 0.2 g

- Saturated Fat 0 g

- Cholesterol 0 mg

- Sodium 18 mg

- Total Carbs 4.1 g

- Fiber 1.3 g

- Sugar 2 g

- Protein 1.2 g

# Strawberry & Spinach Smoothie

## Ingredients

➤ 2 cups fresh spinach

➤ ¾ cup frozen strawberries, sliced

➤ 4–6 drops liquid stevia

➤ 1½ cups unsweetened almond milk

## How to Prepare

1. Add all the ingredients in a high-power blender and pulse until creamy.

2. Pour the smoothie into two glasses and serve immediately.

Preparation time: 10 minutes Total time: 10 minutes Servings: 2

## Nutritional Values

➤ Calories 54

➤ Total Fat 2.9 g

➤ Saturated Fat 0.3 g

- ➢ Cholesterol 0 mg
- ➢ Sodium 159 mg
- ➢ Total Carbs 6.7 g
- ➢ Fiber 2.5 g
- ➢ Sugar 2.8 g
- ➢ Protein 2 g

# Kale & Celery Smoothie

## Ingredients

➤   2 cups fresh kale

➤   1 celery stalk

➤   ½ of avocado; peeled, pitted, and chopped

➤   1 teaspoon fresh ginger, peeled and chopped

➤   1½ cups unsweetened almond milk

➤   ¼ cup ice cubes

## How to Prepare

1.   Add all the  in a high-power blender and pulse until creamy.

2.   Pour the smoothie into two glasses and serve immediately.

Preparation time: 10 minutes Total time: 10 minutes Servings: 2

## Nutritional Values

➤   Calories 170

- ➤ Total Fat 12.5 g

- ➤ Saturated Fat 2.3 g

- ➤ Cholesterol 0 mg

- ➤ Sodium 174 mg

- ➤ Total Carbs 13.7 g

- ➤ Fiber 5.4 g

- ➤ Sugar 0.4 g

- ➤ Protein 3.8 g

# Avocado Smoothie

## Ingredients

➢ 1 large avocado, pitted and sliced

➢ 1 tablespoon fresh lime juice

➢ 1 cup unsweetened almond milk

➢ ½ cup coconut water

➢ ¼ cup ice cubes

## How to Prepare

1. Add all the ingredients in a high-power blender and pulse until creamy.

2. Pour the smoothie into two glasses and serve immediately.

Preparation time: 10 minutes Total time: 10 minutes Servings: 2

## Nutritional Values

➢ Calories 181

➢ Total Fat 16.1 g

- Saturated Fat 3.3 g

- Cholesterol 0 mg

- Sodium 158 mg

- Total Carbs 9.5 g

- Fiber 6.1 g

- Sugar 1.9 g

- Protein 2.3 g

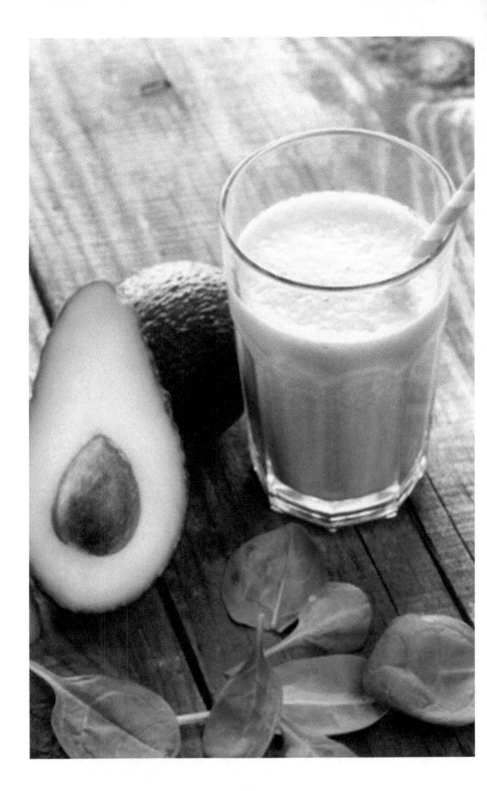

# Cucumber & Parsley Smoothie

## Ingredients

➤ 2 cups cucumber, peeled and chopped

➤ 2 cups fresh parsley

➤ 1 (1-inch) piece fresh ginger root, peeled and chopped

➤ 2 tablespoons fresh lemon juice

➤ 4–6 drops liquid stevia

➤ 2 cups chilled water

## How to Prepare

1. Add all the ingredients in a high-power blender and pulse until creamy.

2. Pour the smoothie into two glasses and serve immediately.

Preparation time: 10 minutes Total time: 10 minutes Servings: 2

## Nutritional Values

➤ Calories 44

- ➢ Total Fat 0.8 g

- ➢ Saturated Fat 0.3 g

- ➢ Cholesterol 0 mg

- ➢ Sodium 39 mg

- ➢ Total Carbs 8.5 g

- ➢ Fiber 2.7 g

- ➢ Sugar 2.6 g

- ➢ Protein 2.7 g

# Grapes Smoothie

## Ingredients

➤ 2 cups seedless green grapes

➤ 1 tablespoon honey

➤ ½ cup fresh apple juice

➤ 1 cup unsweetened almond milk

➤ ¼ cup ice cubes

## How to Prepare

1. Add all the ingredients in a high-power blender and pulse until creamy.

2. Pour the smoothie into two glasses and serve immediately.

Preparation time: 10 minutes Total time: 10 minutes Servings: 2

## Nutritional Values

➤ Calories 196

➤ Total Fat 1.8 g

- ➢ Saturated Fat 0.2 g

- ➢ Cholesterol 0 mg

- ➢ Sodium 96 mg

- ➢ Total Carbs 46.7 g

- ➢ Fiber 1.8 g

- ➢ Sugar 40.2 g

- ➢ Protein 0.6 g

# Kale & Cucumber Smoothie

## Ingredients

- 2 teaspoons green spirulina powder

- 1½ cups fresh kale

- 1 cup cucumber, peeled and chopped

- 1 tablespoon chia seeds

- 1½ cups unsweetened almond milk

- ¼ cup ice cubes

## How to Prepare

1. Add all the ingredients in a high-power blender and pulse until creamy.

2. Pour the smoothie into two glasses and serve immediately.

Preparation time: 10 minutes Total time: 10 minutes Servings: 2

## Nutritional Values

- Calories 84

- ➤ Total Fat 4.1 g

- ➤ Saturated Fat 0.4 g

- ➤ Cholesterol 0 mg

- ➤ Sodium 182 mg

- ➤ Total Carbs 10.7 g

- ➤ Fiber 3.1 g

- ➤ Sugar 0.9 g

- ➤ Protein 4.7 g

# Strawberry, Cucumber & Greens Smoothie

## Ingredients

➤ 1 cup fresh strawberries, hulled and sliced

➤ 1 cup fresh kale, trimmed and chopped

➤ 1 cup fresh spinach, chopped

➤ ½ cucumber, peeled and chopped

➤ 1½ cups unsweetened almond milk

➤ ¼ cup ice cubes

## How to Prepare

1.     Add all the ingredients in a high-power blender and pulse until creamy.

2.     Pour the smoothie into two glasses and serve immediately.

Preparation time: 10 minutes Total time: 10 minutes Servings: 2

## Nutritional Values

➤ Calories 84

➤ Total Fat 3 g

➤ Saturated Fat 0.3 g

➤ Cholesterol 0 mg

➤ Sodium 164 mg

➤ Total Carbs 13.8 g

➤ Fiber 3.4 g

➤ Sugar 4.9 g

➤ Protein 3.2 g

# Kiwi & Banana Smoothie

## Ingredients

➤   1 large frozen banana, peeled and sliced

➤   3 kiwis, peeled and sliced

➤   1 cup fat-free plain yogurt

➤   ½ cup ice cubes

## How to Prepare

1.   Add all the ingredients in a high-power blender and pulse until creamy.

2.   Pour the smoothie into two glasses and serve immediately.

Preparation time: 10 minutes Total time: 10 minutes Servings: 2

## Nutritional Values

➤   Calories 185

➤   Total Fat 0.9 g

➤   Saturated Fat 0.1 g

- Cholesterol 2 mg

- Sodium 90 mg

- Total Carbs 40.7 g

- Fiber 5.2 g

- Sugar 18.6 g

- Protein 7 g

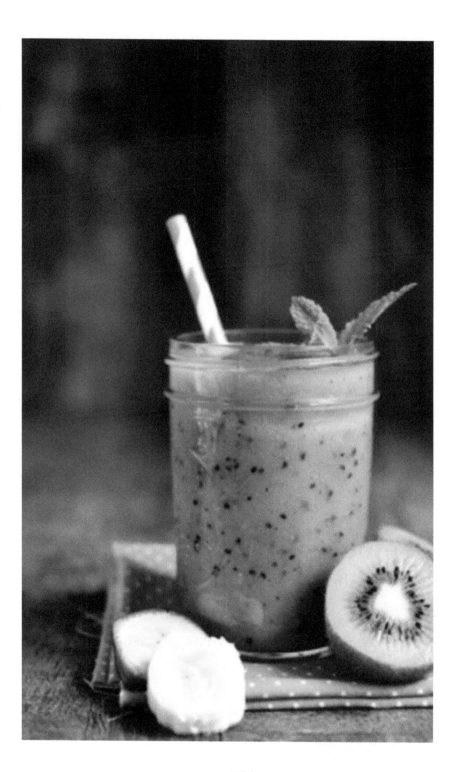

# Green Sunflower Butter Smoothie

## Ingredients

➤ 1 avocado; peeled, pitted, and chopped

➤ 2 cups fresh spinach

➤ 1 scoop unflavored collagen protein powder

➤ 1 tablespoon sunflower seed butter

➤ 1 teaspoon vanilla extract

➤ ½ tablespoon MCT oil

➤ 8–10 drops liquid stevia

➤ 1 cup unsweetened almond milk

➤ 1 cup ice cubes

## How to Prepare

1.    Add all the ingredients in a high-power blender and pulse until creamy.

2.    Pour the smoothie into two glasses and serve immediately.

Preparation time: 10 minutes Total time: 10 minutes Servings: 2

## Nutritional Values

➢ Calories 282

➢ Total Fat 25.8 g

➢ Saturated Fat 7.6 g

➢ Cholesterol 0 mg

➢ Sodium 126 mg

➢ Total Carbs 11.9 g

➢ Fiber 6.9 g

➢ Sugar 0.8 g

➢ Protein 5.6 g

# Cucumber & Mint Smoothie

## Ingredients

➤ 1 large cucumber, peeled and chopped

➤ 1 cup fresh kale

➤ ¼ cup fresh mint leaves

➤ 2 tablespoons fresh lemon juice

➤ 1½ cups unsweetened almond milk

➤ ¼ cup ice, crushed

## How to Prepare

1. Add all the ingredients in a high-power blender and pulse until creamy.

2. Pour the smoothie into two glasses and serve immediately.

Preparation time: 10 minutes Total time: 10 minutes Servings: 2

## Nutritional Values

➤ Calories 78

- ➤ Total Fat 3 g

- ➤ Saturated Fat 0.4 g

- ➤ Cholesterol 0 mg

- ➤ Sodium 159 mg

- ➤ Total Carbs 11.7 g

- ➤ Fiber 2.8 g

- ➤ Sugar 2.8 g

- ➤ Protein 3.2 g

# Creamy Greens Smoothie

## Ingredients

➤    1 cup fresh baby spinach

➤    1 cup fresh baby kale

➤    1 tablespoon almond butter

➤    1 tablespoon chia seeds

➤    1/8 teaspoon ground cinnamon

➤    Pinch of ground cloves

➤    ½ cup heavy cream

➤    1 cup unsweetened almond milk

➤    ½ cup ice cubes

## How to Prepare

1.    Add all the ingredients in a high-power blender and pulse until creamy.

2.    Pour the smoothie into two glasses and serve immediately.

Preparation time: 10 minutes Total time: 10 minutes Servings: 2

## Nutritional Values

➤ Calories 208

➤ Total Fat 18.7 g

➤ Saturated Fat 7.5 g

➤ Cholesterol 41 mg

➤ Sodium 129 mg

➤ Total Carbs 9.1 g

➤ Fiber 3.5 g

➤ Sugar 0.4 g

➤ Protein 5 g

# Cucumber & Lettuce Smoothie

## Ingredients

➤ 1 cucumber, peeled and chopped

➤ 1 cup lettuce leaves

➤ ½ cup fresh mint leaves

➤ 1 tablespoon fresh ginger, grated

➤ 2 cups coconut water

➤ 1 tablespoon fresh lime juice

➤ ¼ cup ice cubes

## How to Prepare

1. Add all the ingredients in a high-power blender and pulse until creamy.

2. Pour the smoothie into two glasses and serve immediately.

Preparation time: 10 minutes Total time: 10 minutes Servings: 2

## Nutritional Values

➢ Calories 92

➢ Total Fat 1 g

➢ Saturated Fat 0.6 g

➢ Cholesterol 0 mg

➢ Sodium 265 mg

➢ Total Carbs 19.1 g

➢ Fiber 5.5 g

➢ Sugar 9.1 g

➢ Protein 3.8 g

Lightning Source UK Ltd.
Milton Keynes UK
UKHW020713270521
384463UK00001B/65